Shared Governan

Beginner

Six Competencies for a Quick Start

By Marsha Parker, RN, BA, MS

MW01038567

Table of Contents

Preface

The emergence of self-published hard copy books and e-books has provided the opportunity for a semi-retired nurse like me to share some of my experience with those of you starting out in a shared governance environment. I had the great good fortune to work with some of the best mentors in shared governance, such as Dr. Tim Porter-O'Grady and Cathleen Wilson, and have helped implement shared governance structures and cultures in multiple organizations. There are a number of really great, professionally done, resources out there for you already. This short book is not meant to compete with any of them. It is a less formal "starter kit" written for the individual to edit and use as they please. Please don't use this book as your only reference, but do use it to help you wade through some of the inevitable confusion of being new to the complexities of shared governance.

It is my hope you can read this book in a relatively short time and develop what will become the groundwork for a very positive growth experience. After more than 50 years in healthcare I can honestly say that my interactions and experiences in shared governance have been the most satisfying and fruitful. I wish the same for you.

Be sure to give me feedback on this guide on my blog at www.EvergreenAuthor.com.

Introduction

Welcome to Shared Governance! This can be one of the most fulfilling journeys you will take as a healthcare employee. It will be what you make of it. Will it be easy? Probably not for some people, but it is definitely doable for everyone and well worth the effort. This book is written to help the beginner get the most out of their initial shared governance (SG) experience and to smooth the sometimes bumpy first steps.

If you are new to healthcare or new to a SG organization you may feel a little put off with having to learn about a completely new structure and philosophy right when you are adapting to a new workplace. Heaven knows healthcare workers are all so busy it can seem pretty daunting to add yet another competency to your practice. You may be hoping you won't have to know very much about it as a new employee and maybe you can just avoid it for a while. Don't let yourself go down that path. In fact, learning the six basic competencies in this book will also help you get oriented in the culture of your new place.

Over the years I have listened to many newcomers as they struggled to get what SG was all about and it is understandable if you would rather ignore the whole thing. You cannot. Don't worry though, you are not alone in feeling as if you have no idea how to start. There will be others just as new as you in your organization and we all have been through that painful beginning. There is help out there. Your organization website likely has the shared governance structure posted and may even have some beginner orientation. Now you have to figure out how to learn it and incorporate it into your own practice.

Hopefully, this guide will help you lay the foundation for not only understanding your role, but help you make your work and practice more fulfilling. In choosing healthcare you already know you have chosen a team approach to your work. There are many specialty paths open to you in the future and whichever one you choose will likely require some work along the way to prepare yourself. Luckily, the skills you learn in SG will help you in almost any job, specialty or role you choose. Critical thinking, problem analysis, team communication and decision making, for example, are useful in everything you will do.

This book is written to help you step through the foundational pieces and get on with the exciting parts of collaborating with your colleagues about the delivery of care and service. The sections are laid out to help you learn the basics and start a plan to learn more. It really can be fun and incredibly satisfying once you wade through the bits and they start making sense as a whole. Pace yourself, but stick with your plan. The result will be that you have a confidence about how to deal in the Shared Governance organization and will, undoubtedly, make wonderful contributions to your patients/clients and your organization.

If you are lucky enough to already have a guide book in your organization use this book as an adjunct to help you clarify and customize a learning plan. Go to the sample learning plan and checklist at the back of this book and on my web site at

www.EvergreenAuthor.com

Copy or print out the Learning Plan and Checklist and start editing them to fit your needs. You can complete everything in them in a week or two if you are a hard charger. A month or two is probably more realistic when you have so much to learn during your orientation and probationary periods.

Keep in mind that **shared governance IS the work** so don't ignore your basic competencies in this part of your practice development.

What is Shared Governance?

"In its simplest form, shared governance is shared decision-making based on the principles of partnership, equity, accountability and ownership at the point of service." (Swihart 2006)

Read more about the principles of shared governance in the references. See "A Note on Resources" section for key links. Dr. Tim Porter-O'Grady's *"Interdisciplinary Shared Governance"* handles the discussion of principles in the first chapter under the heading "Principles for a New Age."

Shared governance moves the control of decisions about the work closer to where the work is done. These decisions become part of your work and part of your practice. Two important things to remember as you learn more about shared governance in your organization.

You cannot abdicate your **responsibility** to support team decisions even if you disagree with them and,

You may take as much **accountability** as you wish in improving outcomes as long as you work through the structure.

Responsibilities are those things that are written in your job description, generally accepted standards and the policies of the organization. Accountabilities are those things that you take on as part of your work or your practice to make things better for your patients, their families or your coworkers. For instance, you must give medications according to the policies of the organization and the professional standard. That is a responsibility. You may make it your accountability to become an expert in managing your diabetic patients and their medications. You may take on the accountability of developing a new process for medication delivery in your unit so there are never any delays. Again, you can take on as much accountability as you wish so long as you work through the structure.

The principle of equity is the one that seems to give beginners the most trouble. Some folks mix up equity and equality. Don't think of Shared Governance as a democracy. It is not a "one man one vote" process for decisions. It doesn't mean every person gets "equal" say in a decision. Instead, those with the most to do with a decision or process have the most say. For instance, a housekeeper will not have much to say about the process of managing a laboring patient, but may have a lot to say about the process of room turnover. The SG approach always tries to bring the right person to the table when their perspective is needed to get the best decision. That is the equity principle. As you are thinking about taking accountability for something don't forget all the other stakeholders involved in that work.

Another place where equity is applied is how work is rewarded. Work is rewarded according to the contribution made. Every person's perspective and contribution are important, but some are more critical to the outcome than others. This is not related to status. Where equity is in play status is not. The culture values every person and every person has access to the rules for team conflict. There is no "lesser" treatment of anyone because of a perceived difference in status.

If you are a "process person" and tend to see work as a series of interrelated processes, then a handy way to view shared governance is as a way for the **stakeholders** of a process to come together and make the best changes to get the best outcomes. The structure of shared governance, like any structure in an organization, is not perfect, but it does allow for more input from the real owners of the work than many other structures. The more engaged you and your coworkers are, the better the decisions about how your work is done.

Competencies for the Beginner

As you develop your learning plan for shared governance take note of some suggested milestones and incorporate them into your plan so you can see your progress. Becoming a member of a shared governance committee can be daunting. It will help you feel more confident of your own knowledge and skills if you have evidence of your initial growth before you consider joining a committee. Check out the tools at the end of this book to make the planning easy.

Some of you are very skilled at creating your own goals and milestones. Please use your critical thinking skills and change or add to the suggestions in this book. At a minimum, consider these competencies:

1. Understand and incorporate the definition and principles of SG into my practice
2. Develop a familiarity with the SG reference and information sources
3. Prepare for and begin the process of engagement in SG
4. Develop SG communication skills
5. Be able to describe the SG structure and how Information flows among the councils
6. Understand the process of SG decision-making

More detailed task are in the checklist and learning plan at the end of this book. Edit them to fit your own needs, but do take the time to complete the contributing tasks and then check them off when you feel more comfortable with each section. Use the nursing process and assess your own progress, diagnose weaknesses in competencies and fix them then reassess. The tools can help you develop your assessment approach. Don't worry about anything being perfect. This is a learning experience and winds up being more art than science. Assess based on how you feel.

Once you feel you are comfortable with the six competencies stop and reassess. You will be ready to move from complete novice to informed novice or intermediate so any weak areas you discover can go into your ongoing development plans.

For longer term development, consider adding, council membership, council leadership (Officer) and teaching a course about shared governance as additional milestones.

The Role of Every Employee in a Shared Governance Environment

You are an owner and stakeholder in shared governance in your organization by virtue of your employment. You may or may not be a primary stakeholder in a particular process or issue being addressed by a committee, but you are a stakeholder. The requirement is that you are an engaged participant and active supporter of the decisions made by teams and committees. If you are a primary stakeholder, then your feedback and input are very important and you should be actively engaged. How do you know if you are a primary stakeholder? Does the decision have impact on your work or your patients? Do you perform the processes that the decision will change? Do you have particular knowledge or expertise about the process? If any of these are true, then you are a primary stakeholder.

Learning about shared governance is something you must do. It is part of your job. It may be outlined in your job description, but, even if it is not, it is a requirement of every employee once administration empowers the shared governance structure to make decisions. Therefore, you must also keep up with the information published by the committees/councils and teams in the structure. That is where you will stay informed about changes and decisions which may influence what you do or how you do it.

Engagement is an inherent part of the role. Engagement is not just participating in a SG governance meeting, it is taking an active, participative interest in how your unit and your organization are operating. Suppose you see a process breakdown like information handoff which could impact patient care or a piece of equipment such as a new IV set that is difficult to use. It is up to you to gather the appropriate information and format it so that it is actionable by the shared governance team or your manager depending on your own structure. Ignoring the problem is not fulfilling the role nor is complaining without providing the information make it actionable. (More about this in Developing Your Voice)

Just as your work is both a team and an individual effort, shared governance is a team effort to make decisions about the team and organizational work while your part as an individual is to engage in the shared decision making and shared leadership to contribute your very best to excellence in service delivery. You are obligated to prepare yourself to act in whatever role you are comfortable, but contribute you must. Engagement is required. How you go about being engaged is up to you.

Once an administration empowers a Shared Governance structure of any kind, the whole organization must support the decisions and actions of the teams and committees. It is not optional. If you are not a nurse and your organization has Nursing Shared Governance, you must support those nursing decisions in whatever way your role allows. It is clearer if you are in an organization which has an integrated structure. However, in either case your obligation as an individual employee is to support the Shared Governance decisions and actions.

If you are not a nurse, you still have the obligation to determine what things decided in shared governance might apply to your own work. Your organization may have whole system shared governance or interdisciplinary shared governance. In that case, anyone may serve on councils and everyone' work will be influenced by the decisions made.

As a professional your role is one of engaged participant and owner. However, as a new person you have time to observe and ask questions. Take a little time and get the lay of the land as long as you don't become a permanent observer.

So how do you "engage" in this early stage? The first step is to prepare yourself with the basics. If you feel prepared you will feel much more comfortable walking into the new situation. There are four things involved in **preparation phase of engagement**:

1. *Educating yourself about the SG structure in your organization.* The unit based structure should be the first one you learn. Find out who serves on that team and introduce yourself. Is there a membership list? Do the positions rotate? How is information distributed?

2. *Learning how to find out what is going on.* Where can you find the agendas of upcoming meetings and the minutes of past meetings which show the decisions which were made? Learn the names of the unit council members. Find out how improvements are being tracked and measured. Are they posted anywhere? Is there a newsletter?

3. *Observing the culture.* How does the environment feel? How do people communicate with one another? Do people feel supported? How are your coworkers engaged?

4. *Keeping your process eyes open.* When you are working notice how things work. Are meds delivered to the units in a timely way? Are they easy to find? Are look-alike meds clearly marked? Do linens arrive in time? Is there enough equipment? Is it hard to get to an open computer? These types of things can impede your work and even endanger patient safety. They are the kinds of things you can help improve along with standards and procedures. See what types of things the unit based SG team is addressing relative to what you have observed.

Once you have prepared yourself with these things then you will be better able to move into the **active engagement phase** with the unit based team.

Your active engagement starts once you see where the team is working and you decide you are ready to jump in there and help. After the review of the minutes from recent meetings and the agenda of the upcoming meeting you may already have some ideas about where you can help. Your mentor, supervisor or SG rep are great people to ask where you best could help.

Keep in mind there are some things that are expected of every actively engaged employee such as working at or above all the standards and expectations for your unit. That means knowing the policies and procedures and understanding the issues your patients and colleagues are dealing with from both clinical and workflow process standpoints.

Additionally, everyone must help the team/s achieve their daily work/performance goals. Know the performance goals and what is being done to achieve them. This may mean, for example, helping a fellow worker in handling the daily workload when he/she is overloaded so that everyone meets the targets. Not only have you helped the team meet goals, you have strengthened the team and the relationships you are building as a new employee. Graciously accepting help can work the same way.

Now, how do you build that active engagement for shared governance specifically?

1. Volunteer to help the unit based *SG team* when you can. Engagement in small things is a great way to learn without being overwhelmed. If you are aware of a new process or procedure the team is testing be sure to support that work by using the new process, volunteering to be part of the test, giving feedback and assisting with measuring and tracking. No need to immediately do anything too complex – you are a novice after all so give yourself a bit of leeway.

2. Research and gather data. When you see a problem or potential problem arise make sure to dig a bit and get some reasons why things

did not go smoothly. Underlying cause is always there waiting for someone to see it. If you don't deal with underlying cause the issue will keep on appearing. It is safe to assume there is a system cause underlying every problem. It is rarely correct to blame a person rather than the process/system. Once you find the underlying causes you can engage with the unit based team to make suggested improvements and avoid future problems. Remember: If you discover a significant safety issue notify your supervisor right away. Safety issues do <u>not</u> wait for team meetings.

3. Communicate. Just chatting with colleagues about the issues the SG team is addressing is a great way to engage and learn. Ask lots of questions. It is also a good way for you to gather information about how others view the work and what they feel is important to them. Practice putting your observations and research about an issue in writing. This takes some time to learn. It is well worth the effort because you will use the skill throughout your career.

A Note on Resources

Hopefully your organization has budgeted time for the work of Shared Governance. Funding a budget which covers the SG meeting times is tough enough these days. There just will never be enough time budgeted/scheduled for all the learning and development of each individual. Take advantage of everything the organization offers, but you will need to go a bit beyond that to develop your own practice. Just as you are accountable for your own professional growth, learning shared decision making and how to present yourself and your issues professionally is your own growth requirement. No matter what your role in the organization you can become an effective presenter of issues and problems along with their possible solutions. This is a significant contribution and constitutes your "voice." More about how to develop an effective voice in shared governance is discussed further on in this book.

There are two reference areas which are SG Beginner "musts." The first is the Shared Governance Forum. There are publications as well as education and networking possibilities for you here. There is a link to an excellent reference titled, "Shared Governance, Third Edition: A Practical

Approach to Inter-Professional Healthcare" by Diana Swihart, PhD and Robert Hess, PhD. Also take a look at Stacey Brull's EASE model infographic. It will give you an easy way to remember basics and works for everyone even if it is geared for nurses.

This site lets you see what is happening in the industry and keep up with some of the latest activities.

http://sharedgovernance.org

The second has been a favorite for many years. Dr. Tim Porter-O'Grady is the Shared Governance guru and has been an invaluable mentor to many of us. He is a prolific writer and has shared his devotion to improving the profession by showing others how to develop expertise in shared governance. This is a place to deepen your knowledge. Please take a look at the site, check out the impressive list of publications and note the free publications you can download from the site.

http://www.tpogassociates.com/

The time you spend getting to know these two sites will be very useful to any beginner in SG and they are full of all sorts of resources. If you want deeper learning, you will appreciate what you can find.

Most shared governance organizations have websites which contain their structures and information about their successes. Some university sites also have free educational materials. These can be very helpful. Just realize that each organization may implement shared governance differently. Surfing around the intranet can be a little confusing if you are expecting shared governance to be standardized across organizations. In fact, there are numerous models and styles of implementation.

Go the site below to read about various models of Shared Governance.

http://www.nursingworld.org/MainMenuCategories/ANAMarketplace/ANAPeriodicals/OJIN/TableofContents/Volume92004/No1Jan04/SharedGovernanceModels.aspx

While this is an older reference it is still very relevant. It is worth the time to read it and it has lots of good references embedded.

Accountabilities of a Shared Governance Beginner

Do I have to be on a committee or a council? This is a common question for beginners. Council membership is a very important contribution to the success of shared governance, but it is not the only way to contribute. Once you have learned the various roles in your unit based team or council and you feel you would not be able to contribute in one of those roles then consider volunteering to help with an improvement project or new procedure implementation and measurement initiated by the council.

Researching the latest literature regarding a particular standard of practice or standards of care may be your preferred place. Maybe you want to help with a social function related to shared governance or develop posters, invitations, newsletters etc. There are many ways to contribute. There are those who feel comfortable as a council member and those who might feel more comfortable in an assistive role. It is really up to you. Ideally, everyone would take a turn serving on a council or one of the action teams/committees assigned by a council to really learn how everything works. In some places the council meetings are open to anyone who wants to attend. Take advantage of this opportunity to get a feel for how things are discussed and determined.

Your organization may have a listing of accountabilities of every employee. If so, please take them seriously. If you are interested you can find listings in websites of other organizations or in some of the SG literature.

Some common accountabilities for individuals include:

1. Empower myself and others
2. Honor the mission of each council in the structure
3. Support decisions of the structure
4. Report problems and issues in actionable format
5. Stay current with team and council actions
6. Inform myself about the facts of an issue before forming an opinion
7. Integrate shared governance competency into my practice growth
8. Participate on a team or council or contribute with my talents
9. Do not demean the work of others even if I do not agree.

10. Do bring opposing opinions to the table when I feel strongly about an issue.
11. *And many more possible accountabilities as chosen by your organization*

Be sure to ask your unit representative if there is a formal listing of these accountabilities.

One of your accountabilities is to learn how to find out what is expected of you in your department. You already know you have to be able to find policies and procedures for your department. That is likely a part of your hospital or unit orientation. There may also be a SG manual or guide book or website to help you learn what is expected of you. Look around the unit for postings and see if there are any newsletters or an archive of newsletters you can read through. If you have a mentor or you have met your SG team representative, you can ask them as well.

The Learning Plan

Start your learning plan now. Pull out the tool and do a quick self-assessment of how you feel when you consider the major items listed? What do you want to learn first? Where are you feeling the least confident? You can change the list any way you want. It is just an example roadmap. If you don't like the plan just use the checklist. Either method will help you get to the destination. The important thing is to just start. Once you are using one of the tools you can see your progress. The checklist could be completed in a week or a couple of months. The speed is up to you. The important thing is to start.

Consider sharing the completed plan or checklist with your mentor, SG rep or supervisor. It will send the message that you are interested in maturing in SG and that you have already developed some groundwork. They will be more likely to think of you as a resource that way.

Developing your "Voice"

Every person in the work place has a valuable perspective (Principle of Equity). Your perspective of how the work is going and how your patients are responding is unique and important. Your understanding of the culture and where there are frustrations and conflict is unique and important. The only issue is that there is a big difference between complaining and offering your perspective. Complaining is negative, often covers only the surface of an issue and is rarely actionable. It leaves a bad feeling with everyone who hears it and can generate conflict. Complaining is about you. Not about the team or the unit. Your "voice" on the other hand is about providing evidence of a process breakdown in such a way that underlying cause is obvious and actionable. This kind of information leaves the listener with a hopefulness that, while there is a problem, there are ways to fix it.

When to use your voice

Newcomers sometimes face the confusion of what types of things to bring up in a shared governance committee. It depends on the committee of course, but since you will be focusing on the unit based team first you will more than likely be talking about issues which effect only your own department. Once the issue has cross departmental impact then other committees or councils come into play. Generally speaking, when in doubt, ask. Experienced team members can quickly guide you to the appropriate place for your issue.

You can legitimately bring up any issue to the SG team, but a cautionary note- any issue which might cause an immediate safety issue for your co-workers, visitors or patients must be taken immediately to your supervisor. Safety issues are dealt with immediately and do not wait for any group to meet. When in doubt about these types of problems go to your supervisor.

Issues typically fall into a couple of categories, clinical issues and workflow issues. There are usually procedures in place to deal with personal conflicts, but those are not usually brought to a SG team. Instead look for issues that obstruct or restrict the very best in clinical care. Are the standards not up to date for the specific patient load on your unit? Is there a logistics issue with supplies or medications distribution? Could there be an improvement on communications about transitions of care to or from your area or during discharge? Are the education materials you are using in need of update? Are the policies unclear? Anything like this can be a good issue for the shared governance team. They will let you know if it should be taken elsewhere.

Why won't they listen?

Suppose you have taken an issue to the team and they don't put it on the agenda or they don't have discussion about it? There are a number of reasons to consider. Have you provided enough information for the issue to be actionable or is someone having to do more work before the issue can be put on the agenda? Has this issue been discussed before? Are other issues taking priority over yours? It is worth taking the time to ask a team member about the status of your issue. Don't be put off if the council doesn't immediately put your issue as the next newsletter headline. Just patiently work through the obstacles. This is a golden learning opportunity.

The most frequent cause of an issue not making the agenda is the lack of enough information to make the issue actionable. Go to the Tools section at the end of the book to see a couple of tools which may help you create issue documentation which will get your voice heard.

A few things to remember. Get opinions from others on your unit. Gather data about the issue and evidence of the problems the issue causes. You might show the process in a flow chart and highlight the problem areas. Root out and document underlying causes. Suggest some solutions. Do not name names or lay blame.

One of the most important things to keep in mind is to be gracious no matter what the decision is regarding your issue. If it is not heard immediately, do try to bring it forward again later after you have some feedback. Just because it isn't on the agenda for the next meeting doesn't mean it won't eventually be there. If the decision doesn't go the way you had hoped, stay positive and support the decision that was made. In the long run this attitude will gain you the willingness of the team to listen to the next issue you bring up. Hang in there and keep learning.

How to make them want to listen.

It is an art, not a science. The most important thing is to be as clear as possible and be able to back up your assertions with evidence. Check with your SG rep to see if there is a format approved by the team or councils to use for bringing and issue forward. If so, please use that. If there is not an approved format you can use the one in the Tools section of this book. Whatever you do, remember what it is like to be very busy and to have only a precious hour or two to get through an issue and make a decision.

Presenting to a team can be done in person or in writing. Please do both. If you are presenting in person send your handouts ahead of time so the members can read them before the meeting. Even if you have a PowerPoint presentation it is a good idea to send a copy of the presentation and any handouts ahead of time so team members have time to peruse them before the meeting.

Start with an executive summary which outlines everything in a page or so. Then have your data, process, causes, outcomes and solutions documented in the following sheets. Make everything as clear as possible. In this day and age there is no reason pictures cannot be added to your documents to clarify if necessary. Use diagrams or process maps to help show the exact steps causing the issue. If you have conducted interviews with others use a table showing opinions, but don't quote each individual specifically unless the quote is critical to understanding the issue. If the chair is interested in exactly who was interviewed you can provide the list privately. Otherwise, just identify the numbers and roles of those providing information

How Decisions Are Made In Shared Governance

Decisions in shared governance teams are one of the stumbling blocks for the newcomer. You probably have a lot of experience with decisions made by the manager or supervisor or, perhaps, by your instructors. You may also be used to an elected leader of a team making the decisions. In a shared governance council or team all the perspectives are brought together, discussed and a group consensus reached. This does NOT mean everyone has to agree. In fact, there are often those who do not agree with one decision or another, but who still support the decision of the group. Another time it may be them receiving the support from others. That is not to say the team leader or council chair cannot make a decision and often must do so when an immediate answer is needed. However, the lead/chair must then bring that decision to the next team meeting and explain why that particular decision was made.

The most frequently made mistake is to simply dump a problem on the team. Often SG team members are used as the place to complain about something that isn't working and then the complainer walks away thinking the responsibility for solutions is now belongs to the council. That is simply not the case. In shared governance the person bringing the issue forward retains the responsibility to track the issue and support any solutions. It is not that you have to solve every problem and implement yourself, but you do have support your SG team as they deal with the issue. Your team will be much more likely to believe you are serious about problems getting resolved if you are part of the solution.

To create a competency in decision-making, start with critical thinking about an issue. Learning to listen carefully is step number one. You must fully understand the issue and its underlying causes before you can select the best solution option. Step number two is to make sure you have heard from the various stakeholders. Hopefully, the issue presenter will have interviewed and documented the input from the stakeholders. Remember that principle of Equity? Don't limit the input for an issue to a select group with which you feel comfortable. Elicit opinions from someone in each role connected to the issue whether they are positive or negative. Step number three is to collaboratively discuss the options while considering the impact the options have on other roles and departments.

Now comes the hard part. It is not always that the majority rules. It is the weight of the key stakeholders which can sway a decision. If there are a couple of experts in the discussion and they are strongly in agreement that a particular option is the best then the rest of the group may have to decide if their feeling are strong enough to counter those of the experts. Each council has its own personality and will interpret the "weight" of opinion differently. Here is the comforting codicil. In the long run the justice of this approach becomes more and more refined. People become more cautious about swaying a decision overly much because they are living with the results of those decisions and the results are very apparent to peers. It really does lean toward balance over time.

Understanding the Shared Governance Structure

In a shared governance structure or shared leadership structure the old vertical lines of authority do not exist. Decisions and outcomes are owned by the staff. Because collaboration and partnership replace the old authority role the structures often look like circles and because the focus is on the point of service the unit based councils are often portrayed as the center of the structure. The groups defined in the structure can vary so be sure to check your own organization's structure, but here are the basics.

The groups are usually called councils, but can also commission action committees or project teams so don't get lost in the terminology. The organization-wide councils address issues that apply to multiple departments. Things like education, quality, practice/standards, multidepartment process issues and management would be addressed by these councils. There is usually an organization wide coordinating or governance council which deals with keeping the structure working effectively and with issues affecting more than one council. Some typical councils might be:

1. Unit based Councils
2. Practice and Standards Council
3. Education Council
4. Quality Council
5. Coordinating Council
6. Management or Operations Council
7. Service Council
8. ET. Al.

If your organization is just starting with SG you may also have some sort of Initiating Committee or Council the charter of which includes the fostering of the SG culture and structure through its infancy. Most often this group goes away once things are up and running.

Information sharing among the councils and out to their constituents is always difficult because of the time constrictions for healthcare workers. There is usually a publishing of agendas before meetings so all employees can see what is to be discussed and another publishing of the minutes after the meetings. These may be electronic posting on an organization's intranet or a paper newsletter. Most of the organization-wide meetings are monthly or less while the unit based councils may meet weekly so there is not a lot of time for person to person communication. Some things may be brought up in department meetings or posted in communication books which you read an initial.

If the timing of communications create a problematic delay then the chair of the first council can meet with the chair of the second council to see how the issue could be handled in a more timely way. That may result in the chair making a decision or the chair assigning some members to be a decision group. In the last couple of examples the chair must present the decision to the entire council at the next meeting and explain why the decision had to be made quickly.

Sometimes the communications among councils are handled by having a list of final decisions circulated to all councils. Another way is to have members sit on two councils – one being the home council and one being the role of communicator between councils. Check out how it is done in your organization.

Rules of Communication

A better title might be the Civilities of Communication in Shared Governance. There may or may not be written rules about how your organization expects interactions to be handled. But consider this. If the principles include partnership and equity then understanding how to incorporate those principles in communications will help foster the partnerships. Other types or styles which may be more confrontational or aggressive may not engender partnership. Hammering home your individual opinion without collaboration just doesn't work in this environment. Even if the person making the demands is absolutely right the long term effect of high tension, unilateral communications will not gain willing partners. That is not to say you cannot be assertive. There is a difference as you know.

Some unwritten rules:

- If there is conflict two rules apply. Intervene, then get to the origin of the conflict and create a safe place for the resolution discussions. Listening and calm questions help deescalate the tensions. Do not let conflict expand into a political uproar. Animated discussion of varying views is fine. Hurtful conflict is not.
- Think of all communications as a means to connect or reconnect. That means think about your wording and assume everyone in the organization will read or hear it.
- Be complete, but not overly wordy. It is true a picture is worth a thousand words.
- Don't demean anyone else or their work in any of your communications.
- Don't show a preference for one option over another until the collaborative discussion.
  This is a form of lobbying before the meeting.
- When communicating a decision with which you do not agree, do not start out by saying, "I don't agree with this, but….." Support the decision as if you agree with it.
- Don't presume authority over any other attendee of a council when you are speaking about an issue. If you are an RN and an aide is speaking or you are responding to an opinion from an aide both opinions have value and are not connected to the status of a title. The same is true for a physician attendee or member. The physician, like everyone else, must leave status at the door.
- Wait until someone else is done before speaking.
- Stop and think about a person's statements before responding.
- Never be accusing or blaming in communications.

You can probably think of another dozen or so unwritten rules. Recall any time you were made uncomfortable by a style or tone of communication. Those have to be avoided in shared governance in order to foster the collaborative culture. The true test is when you can be a reasoned communicator in the face of overly forceful, loud or blaming opponents.

Some new members may feel as if the councils are not well supported by administration or their own manager and wonder if it is a bad thing to get involved in shared governance. Thankfully, this is not a common occurrence. However, if you do run into it, consider this. The skills you learn will be with you throughout your career whether that particular manager is or not. The relationships you build with your colleagues is a professional network which is a benefit anyplace you might work and stays with you personally, not the organization. Lastly, work satisfaction comes from having a voice in how the work is done. If you abdicate your role as owner what other role would you like to have?

New Council Members

If you are relatively new to SG and you have been asked to join a council, or if you just want to be prepared to join, there are a few must do tasks.

Get your hands on any written materials such as a charter or mission statement, minutes and agendas and any whitepapers or issues documents as soon as you can. Go back at least six months. If your council has a blog read the postings back several months. The purpose is that you don't go into the first meeting cold and then asked your opinion when there has already been tons of discussion about that very issue. You won't then be in a place where you are proposing solutions which have already been ruled out.

In that same vein it is important to talk with a couple of other members of the council and ask them about hot topics or difficult recent meetings. Ask them to help you understand how the group works and how they feel about the performance of the group to date. Be sure to ask them of what they are most proud.

When you know the upcoming issues don't be content to just read them. Educate yourself about them. Read the literature and get some best practice background, ask coworkers their opinions and think through some possible organizational obstacles. Can you observe those obstacles in action? A bit of work on your part will really show when you are in the meeting. You will be able to determine if the presenter of an issue has done a thorough job of preparing or not and you will know what questions to ask. Bring references with you in case someone else might be interested in learning more.

Keep up with what is on the agendas of other councils. It often happens that someone will bring something up and, rather than spending precious discussion time on something already being discussed elsewhere you can create an information link to the other council for your next meeting.

Yes, a picture is worth a thousand words. So are process maps, timelines and diagrams. There is a whole science out there about these types of things. You may have seen some of the work of your Quality Department in process maps and Pareto Charts. That is not, necessarily, what this is about. Sure, if you have those skills be sure to use them. However, this is about using pictures, hand drawings on a white board, charts or other graphics to illustrate an issue and facilitate a clearer discussion. This is about the art of communication. If you are going to present an issue or problem to the council you should be able to get all the information needed for the group to make a decision or take an action in one meeting. You can expect to have others read your materials before the meeting. That, of course, requires you to have submitted your materials in time. Find out what that timing is for meeting preparation. Don't forget you must also read all the materials that come to you from other presenters.

Take a look at the issue preparation document at the end of this book or go to www.evergreenauthor.com to copy or print. Feel free to edit. You can print the WORD or PDF form. It is meant to be a help as you develop the issue information for presentation. Your organization may already have one of these forms so be sure to ask the council secretary.

Communicating to constituency is part of the role of all council members. How that is done is different in every structure or model of SG. Be sure to know the expectation before you leave the first meeting. Your target audience, the methods of communication and the timeline for communicating are all important elements to know. Some places use all electronic postings of information to the stakeholders and others use fliers, handouts or communication books.

If you are assigned to attend other council meetings as a liaison from your own council be sure you understand what kinds of things you should report and what kinds of things you should bring back. It would be embarrassing to get there and find out they expect a formal report of activities and outcomes when you are not prepared. Sometimes there is a discussion of successes and failures or just a sharing of final decisions and the implications. You just need a heads up before you go. Generally, the collegial sharing in these settings is very interesting and satisfying.

A Note to Scholars

Those of you who are serious about nursing research or just love the use of analytics and data, please add your own level of sophistication to the basics in this book. If you have the presentation skills or project management skills already, then, please, use them to help raise the standards of communication and practice improvement in your organization. You have something extra to add to the mix when it comes to decision making.

Consider helping a colleague add data and presentation polish to their own offering. Helping a colleague succeed in voicing a problem and then having the team choose to implement the recommended solution can be a career changer and a terrific boost to their confidence. Who knows how many other problems that person will help solve over the years because you chose to help?

Tools To Help You Learn And Improve Your Shared Governance Practice.

It is outside the scope of this book to go into detail about the use of each tool. That will be in another book in this series. However, the tools listed here and on the website are pretty simple and you can likely figure them out on your own or with the descriptions below. Formatting is not great on tablets so the contents of the tools are also shared here. The scanned versions of the tools are attached in the appendix. If you want to edit the tool or do some of your own formatting then go to the website mentioned below where you can find the WORD versions. They are yours to do with as you wish.

The first toolkit in this section is the learning plan or checklist. You can use either or both. Their purpose is to give you a clear picture of your progress and help your confidence as you begin to actively engage in shared governance activities.

The second toolkit contains data collection and presentation tools for you to use in both a practice exercise as well as an actual presentation of an issue to a council. These are the tools for expressing an issue to your supervisor, a team or a council. Use them to develop your professional voice for these interactions.

Preparing a documented issue ready for action takes a little bit of work. To save you time and effort three tools have been included with this book. The first is a process investigation sheet. The second is a data collection tool and the last is a presentation format for you to use to present the issue to a council. The tools may be helpful, but they are certainly not required. If you feel confident in your data collection, analysis and presentation skills you can skip this part.

Shared Governance Learning Toolkit

Print out the tool and fill it out as you complete each step. You may want to share it with your SG rep so he/she knows you are prepared to assist with some of the work of the Unit Committee or Council.

Here are the contents. A scanned version is in the Appendices. A WORD version form with checkboxes is available at

www.evergreenauthor.com.

Overall Goal: To achieve beginning competencies and prepare to actively engage in the work of shared governance.

Pre Assessment: How comfortable am I with:

1. What shared governance is and its basic principles?
2. Where to find references and internal information sources?
3. How to prepare for and then actively engage in unit based SG activities?
4. How to put together a documented issue so your voice can be heard?
5. What each council does and how they interact?
6. How decisions are made in the structure?

Competency 1: Understand the definition and principles of shared governance.

A. Definition
B. Partnership
C. Equity
    a. Differences between equity and equality
    b. Equity in decision making
D. Accountability
    a. Differences between accountability and responsibility
    b. Personal accountabilities of employees in this organization
E. Ownership

Competency 2: References and information sources.

A. Minutes and agendas of the unit based council meetings
B. Minutes and agenda sources for all other SG councils/committee
C. Find your organization's websites or postings.
D. Go out to the two major links recommended
E. Read the article regarding models

Competency 3: Engagement

A. Preparation
    a. Learned the structure and how information flows from one council to another
    b. Observed the cultural aspects:
        i. Sharing and support
        ii. Conflict and frustrations; status and what it means
        iii. Groups and cliques
        iv. How informed are co-workers about SG activities
B. Active Engagement
    a. Volunteered to help
    b. Discussed agenda items and decisions with coworkers
    c. Attended a meeting or meetings to observe.
    d. Implemented decision results in your own practice and offered feedback

Competency 4: Communication and "Voice"

A. Documented a sample issue using the tool
B. Showed my example to a coworker for feedback
C. Learned and incorporated rules of communication

Competency 5: Structure and Information Flow

A. Can describe the councils in my structure including the mission/charter of each
B. Can describe how information flows from council to council

Competency 6: Decision Making

A. I understand equity and collaboration in decision making
B. I support all decisions of the councils/committees even when I disagree with them.
C. Am familiar with the issue documentation and presentation tools in this book.

Post-assessment:
Following the steps above how comfortable am I with:
1. What shared governance is and its basic principles?
2. Where to find references and internal information sources?
3. How to prepare for and then actively engage in unit based SG activities?
4. How to put together a documented issue so your voice can be heard?
5. What each council does and how they interact?
6. How decisions are made in the structure?

Continuing and Future Learning Goals:

1.

2.

End of form

Issue Presentation Toolkit
Preparing a documented issue ready for action takes a little bit of work. To save you time and effort three tools have been included with this book. The first is a process investigation sheet. The second is a data collection tool and the last is a presentation format for you to use to

present the issue to a council. Go to the website below to print out or download WORD formatted tools.

www. evergreenauthor.com

The first tool in this toolkit allows you to list the steps in the process which have broken or to the show why it is not working effectively. Just list the detailed steps of the process in chronological order and note any delays or errors, breakdown points or failure points in the process. Now ask a person doing the work to give you their thoughts about why the process breaks down. The rule of thumb is to ask, "Why?" five times to try to get to the underlying cause. If you can get two or three people who do the work to fill out this sheet your data process information will be pretty reliable. This is a worksheet. Don't worry if it gets messy because you will summarize it anyway.

Contents of the Process Investigation Sheet:
Name and Department

Process Being Described

The main part of the Investigation requires the person list each task in the process. For each task include the following information. These are good headers and work well in an Excel format or a WORD table.

Number of the Task, Brief Description of the Task, Is this a Failure Point? What Kind of Failure? Underlying Cause

The formatted tool has five symbols with a key at the bottom of the sheet. These are optional. The benefit of using them is that together they form a process map. The symbols are: action/task, delay, question, purge and document. They help you see how this process might be related to other processes. For instance, was a document generated at specific step? Does this document generate other actions? If you delete it will it mean an important action does not happen?

You may want to specify where the process investigation starts and stops. Do this by writing a starting task at the top of the page in the first task slot. Then ask those helping you to write all the steps from that task until the place you want to stop.

The second tool is just for data collection and your own notes. The most difficult thing to decide is what to measure. At a minimum you will need the number of times an incident/breakdown has occurred in the last few weeks or months. If you can measure the outcome which resulted from the breakdown then by all means collect that information. For instance, eight patients had medication delays, six had no harm, but were frustrated with the delays and two had to have an intervention.

Contents of the Data Collection Tool

Section One: A description of the problem and any goals you have for your project

Section Two: The measures of the problem. Typically, how often does it occur and how many times have there been outcomes of various sorts. You can even measure near misses. Interviews can also be a measure.

Section Three: A spreadsheet or listing of the actual data including the related dates and roles if you are listing interview results. Include a column for notes related to each item.

Section Four: Failure point information from process maps or the Process Investigation Sheets.

Section Five: A summary of the above information, your analysis and any underlying causes

Section Six: Conclusions and recommendations.

The third tool outlines a simple method of presenting an issue which you can fill in and then provides a way to display the data you have collected. Of course the most effective method includes graphs of your data and even pictures – especially if your issue involves less than ideal equipment. However, fancy is not required. Clarity is. Try it out. See if you can use these tools to document a sample issue in your area and then ask a coworker to read it to see if they could make a decision based on what you have provided.

Contents of a Presentation Tool

Section One: Summary of the problem, brief description of findings of the investigation and recommendations for resolution. No more than one page.

Section Two: Presentation of your method of investigation and the results. Include graphics if applicable. Explain why particular measures were used.

Section Three: Your analysis and conclusions. Include a summary map if applicable. Up to and including this section the presentation is about the current practice.

Section Four: Can be more than one option. Discuss how you collaborated to develop the options. Discuss the roles of the stakeholders involved in this process and how their interested are represented.

Conclusion and Encouraging Words

Now that you have read through this short book and completed either the checklist or the learning plan do you feel a little less confused about:

7. What shared governance is and its basic principles?
8. Where to find references and internal information sources?
9. How to prepare for and then actively engage in unit based SG activities?
10. How to put together a documented issue so your voice can be heard?
11. What each council does and how they interact?
12. How decisions are made in the structure?

As you complete your reassessment ask yourself if you feel more ready for your initial foray into SG, but don't set the expectation that you will be supremely confident as if you are an expert. You have plenty of time to get to that level. Take the first step or two and see how things go. There will be colleagues to assist you along the way. Remember you started from knowing nothing. Take the time to celebrate your early progress.

The six competencies covered in this book are not enough to make you a huge SG success in the first couple of months you are in a SG environment, but they definitely will get you off to a good start.

Hopefully, this guide has helped you avoid some of the trickier issues and confusing bits beginners often face as they orient to shared governance.

Even this short book can seem like a lot at first, but it will all come together as you gain more experience with the shared governance process. Just keep in mind that healthcare needs the voice of every single stakeholder and you now have an avenue for your contributions. Make the most of it and look back at your work in shared governance knowing the value of your participation.

If you have questions or feedback about anything in this book, please feel free to ask them on my blog at

www.evergreenauthor.com

I would love to hear if the book helped or how it might be made better. You can leave your reviews at Amazon.com as well.

References

Anthony, M. K. (2004) "Shared governance models: The theory, practice and evidence". Online Journal of Issues in Nursing, http://nursingworld.org/oijn/topic23/tpc23_4.htm

Porter-O'Grady, T. (2009) *Interdisciplinary share governance: Integrating practice, transforming healthcare*. Jones and Bartlett Publishers, Sudbury, MA, 01776.

Swihart, D. (2006) *Shared governance: A practical approach to reshaping Nursing practice*. HCPro Inc. Marblehead, MA 01945

Links:

Shared Governance Forum http://sharedgovernance.org

Dr. Tim Porter-O'Grady and Associates http://www.tpogassociates.com/

Author website where you can find the tools www.evergreenauthor.com

Appendices:

Figure 1: The Learning Plan (pgs1-3)

Shared Governance Quick Start Learning Plan

Name:		
Role/Title:		
Date Started:		✅
Check off items	Notes of Accomplishment	Completed?
Overall Goal: To achieve beginning competencies and prepare to actively engage in the work of shared governance.		
Pre-Assessment – Understanding of the 6 competencies: 1. Definitions and principles 2. Information sources 3. Engagement 4. Communication and voice 5. Structure and info flow 6. Decision making	Overall 1. 2. 3. 4. 5. 6.	Overall 1. 2. 3. 4. 5. 6.
Competency 1: Understanding the definition and principles of shared governance.	*What is it?*	
Definition		
Partnership		
Equity		
- Differences between equity and equality		
- Equity in decision making		
Accountability		
- Differences between accountability and responsibility		
- Personal accountabilities of employees in this organization		
Ownership		
Competency 2: References and information sources.	*Where I found them.*	
Minutes and agendas of the unit based council meetings		
Minutes and agenda sources for all other SG councils/committee		
Find your organization's websites or postings.		
Go out to the two major links recommended		
Read the article regarding models		
Competency 3: Engagement	*What I did and what I observed.*	
Preparation		
Learned the structure and how information flows from one council to another – also see Competency #5		
Observed the cultural aspects:		
- Sharing and support		
-Conflict and frustrations; status sources		

Page 2

Check off items	Notes of Accomplishment	Completed?
-Groups and cliques		
-How informed co-workers are about SG activities		
Active Engagement		
Volunteered to help		
Discussed agenda items & decisions with coworkers		
Attended meetings to observe		
Competency 4: Communication and "Voice"	*How have I communicated?*	
Documented a sample issue using the tool.		
Showed my example to a coworker to see if they understood the information		
Learned and incorporated the rules of communication.		
I shared the results of the Unit Based Council with others		
Competency 5: Structure and Information Flow		
Councils in the structure are:	*Their Missions/Charters are located:*	
Unit Based Council		
Practice Council		
Mgmt/Operations Council		
Education Council		
Quality Council		
Governance/Coordinating		
Service Council		
Information shared from Council to Council is:	*Which way does it flow?*	

MP/version 3/2015

Page 3

Competency 6: SG Decision-Making	Give examples	
I understand equity in decision-making		
I understand collaboration in decision-making		
I support all decisions of the councils/committees even when I disagree with them.		
I have observed decisions being made in the SG structure.		
Post-Assessment – Understanding of the 6 competencies: 1. Definitions and principles 2. Information sources 3. Engagement 4. Communication and voice 5. Structure and info flow 6. Decision making	Overall 1. 2. 3. 4. 5. 6.	Overall 1. 2. 3. 4. 5. 6.
Learning Goals for Continued Development 1. 2. 3, 4. 5.		
Comments:		
Completed this checklist on: (Date) Signature:		

MP/version 3/2015

3

Figure 2: The Checklist

Shared Governance for Beginners Checklist

#	Task or Learning Item	Date Completed
1	Completed the pre-assessment	
2	Learn what shared governance is.	
3	Understand the principles of:	
	• Ownership	
	• Partnership	
	• Equity	
	• Accountability and difference from responsibility	
4	Found the following:	
	• Minutes and agendas of unit based council	
	• Minutes and agendas of other councils	
	• My institutions website and SG references	
	• Any guidebooks	
	• Any SG Org charts, mission statements or charters	
	• List of names of members of my unit council	
	• Other?	
5	Learned the structure and what each council does as well as how information flows among them	
6	Went to web and found the two main reference sites:	
	• Forum for Shared Governance – http://sharedgovernance.org	
	• Dr. Porter-O'Grady site – http://tpogandassociates.com	
7	Found and read the Shared Governance Models article	
8	Completed culture observations for:	
	• Sharing and support of each other	
	• How conflict and frustrations are handled	
	• Who has status and why	
	• What groups and cliques are there	
	• How informed others are about SG activities	
9	Volunteered to help with	
	•	
	•	
10	Discussed upcoming unit based agenda items with coworkers	
11	Documented a sample issue using the tool and got feedback	
12	Understand "equity" in decision making and my role as stakeholder	
13	Understand that I support all decisions of the council even if I disagree.	
14	Completed the post assessment	
Future learning tasks:		
Signature:		

Figure 3: The Process Information Collection Tool

Process: _____   *Symbols are optional*

#	Tasks in Chronological Order	Avg Time	Failure Point?	■	▲	▣	◆	●	Possible Underlying Causes
1									
2									
3									
4									
5									
6									
7									
8									
9									
10									
11									
12									
13									
14									
15									
16									
17									
18									
19									
20									

Investigator Name: _____

■ Action/Task   ▲ Delay   ▣ Document   ◆ Question   ● Purge   ⟋ Draw connector lines   Page #_____

Figure 4: Data Collection Tool

Use this tool to document what you find as you investigate an issue. Then convert the information to presentation format. If this is an incident this form does NOT replace an incident report in your facility reporting system.

Investigator Name:

Describe the issue. Do not use the phrases, "What is needed or We need..." That would be a solution statement which you use later in your recommendations. This is a description of the failure or breakdown.	Date range of observations or interviews	Is this an immediate threat to safety? *If "yes" report to supervisor immediately.*

Goal/s of this project: Such as reduce the # of breakdowns by x %.

Process steps where breakdown occurred: Write in text or draw out the steps. You can insert a Visio or PowerPoint drawing here. Use the failure points you discovered using the process tool

Number of times in XX days the breakdown occurred.		Underlying Causes of Breakdowns sorted by greatest cause first.
Severity of the breakdown/s and impact on patient		1.
1.		2.
2.		3.
3.		4.
Comments:		5.
Interviewee Name & Role	Results	6.
1 Date		7.
		8.
2 Date		Comments and Notes:
3 Date		

1

Page 2

Observations or Measures:				
Steps observed	Findings	Measures	Findings/ Comments	Date and Time

Summary of all findings above:

Analysis of above - Determine areas requiring immediate focus or areas most likely to result in greatest improvement

Options for Improvement and recommendations

Figure 5: Presentation Tool

Summary Page:

Problem

Scope and impact of the problem

Summary of investigation findings

Options and recommendations

Page 2

Shared Governance Issue Presentation Tool

Detailed Findings of Current State:

Problem Statement: Include the details of frequency, duration and severity about the problem demonstrating the current state

Include any graphics, summary interview findings and observations in this section which will help the reader understand the problem. Do not include every detail of your investigation. Illustrate – don't frustrate. If they are easily understood you can include spreadsheets. This may take several pages depending on the issue.

Description of Analysis: Brief description of methods you used to get to underlying cause and how you prioritized findings and recommendations.

Discussions with Stakeholders re: Future State: Include enough so that the group is clear about how you collaborated to come up with some of the options for resolution.

Options for Resolution: Include two or three of the best option, why they are the best and even the pros and cons of each if it will help the group come to a decision. Use as much space as you need to make the options clear.

Option One	Pros	Cons
Option One	Pros	Cons
Option One	Pros	Cons

Notes and Comments:

Made in the USA
San Bernardino, CA
25 January 2020

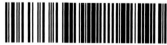

63617263R00024